What Is Beta Glucan?

- Immunity
- Cholesterol
- Tumors
- Blood sugar
- Skin rejuvenation

by

Roger Mason

WHAT IS BETA GLUCAN?

A Concise Guide to the Benefits and Uses of the Most Powerful Natural Immune Enhancer Known to Science

by

Roger Mason

What Is Beta Glucan?
by
Roger Mason

Copyright 2001 by Roger Mason

What is Beta Glucan?
by
Roger Mason

ISBN #1-884820-66-2
Printed in the U.S.A.

Safe Goods/New Century Publishing 2000
60 Bullock Dr., Unit 6   PO Box 36
Markham, ON L3P 3P2   East Canaan, CT 06024
(905) 471-7885   (888) 628-8731

Contents

About This Book

Beta glucan has been known to scientists as a plant constituent for decades. For over twenty years now it has been studied for the favorable biological effects on mammals. It has been common knowledge in the scientific community that beta glucan is the most powerful immune stimulant known, is a very powerful antagonist to both benign and malignant tumors, lowers cholesterol and triglycerides, normalizes blood sugar levels, heals and rejuvenates the skin and has various other benefits.

Yet in 2001 no one has bothered to write a book on the subject. There have been a couple of incomplete attempts to write small pamplets that merely skim the surface. Go ahead and search the Internet for anything on "beta glucan" and see what you get. Search amazon.com and barnes&noble.com and you'll get the same result. I went back to 1980 in the main scientific reference journal of the world Chemical Abstracts- the "Scientists Bible"- and went over every listing for the last 21 years. Every relevant abstract was copied, every important study was obtained and translated from foreign languages if necessary. All these were collated and put together in to this easy to read, plain English short book. Why not, say, a 200 page book? Because that was unnecessary and most people just aren't going to take the time to read a long book. All you need to know is in here. Everything you need to know and more is in this short book. It won't take you long at all to read it, and after you read it I hope you'll decide to take beta glucan for the rest of your life like I have. This is one of the most important supplements you can take to be healthy, have strong immunity and live a long life.

You'll notice there are no companies recommended, phone numbers or addresses or any brand names listed. Products and companies change all the time so find the best brand at the best price wherever you can.

Roger Mason
Summer 2001

Overview

This is a factual book. It is also a very thoroughly documented book replete with dozens and dozens of published scientific references. You may find it a little dry at times but there is a reason for this- my only intent is to document the scientific studies that show the amazing power of this natural supplement.

I find that the natural supplement industry is, like all other industries, basically directed towards advertising and profits. You hear endless promotions for various supplements that claim to do miraculous things for your health and cure your ills. Many of these natural supplements are, in fact, very powerful and effective while remaining very safe and non-toxic. For the layman it becomes impossible to separate fact from fiction since these promotions are so skillfully and professionally written. In the case of beta glucan one company swears only yeast glucan is valid, while another swears only oat glucan is effective, while a third swears that only mushroom glucan works. You'll see here that all true 1,3 beta glucans work regardless of their source.

This book was written objectively and factually with no profit motive. After reading these six chapters you should agree that beta glucan is one of the most important supplements you can take. You'll see that beta glucan is the most powerful immunity enhancer known to science. Beta glucan is now being used on real people with cancer to see how it can assist in other therapies. You will especially want to try taking beta glucan if you suffer from malignancies, high cholesterol, a weak immune system, or diabetes. Healthy people will want to take it to become even stronger and feel better.

It has only been in the last two years that technology has brought the price down to where we can get potent 100 mg and 200 mg capsules very inexpensively, as well as real topical creams with an honest 1% glucan content. This has been known about for over 20 years but the extraction technology didn't make this practical and inexpensive for the general public until 1999. Take advantage of this and make it a part of your daily supplement program.

Chapter 1: What Is Beta Glucan?

Beta glucan is a polysaccharide (i.e. "many sugars", a chain of glucose molecules) that is found in such foods as oats, barley, mushrooms and yeasts. Beta glucan has been known to scientists as a food constituent for decades, and they knew it was abundant in the foods as just named. It is extremely difficult to extract and purify, however. Oat bran contains about 15% beta glucan and is inexpensive but hard to use at such low strength for oral capsules or skin lotions. It wasn't until the 1980's that commercial beta glucan creams started appearing and they were very weak- too weak to be effective due to the still very high cost of extracting it. Finally a few years ago, about 1999 technology succeeded in producing less expensive beta glucan from both oats and brewers yeast (after the beer was brewed). Now oral capsules were offered in amounts that were honestly biologically effective and a few good topical creams appeared.

Some companies, however, heavily advertised their products but still refused to put realistic amounts of beta glucan in their supplement. One company, for example, put out two different strengths- one was called "-24" but only actually contained a mere 3 mg of beta glucan per capsule. The other was called "-100" but only actually contained a mere 10 mg and was very, very expensive. Both were therefore useless biologically despite extensive advertising and a temporary success in the marketplace. Another sold a product with only 7.5 mg in each capsule for a very high price. Fortunately other companies came out with 100 mg, 250 mg and even 500 mg capsules so people could get the benefits the clinical studies got in test animals.

During the year 2000 even further breakthroughs happened and beta glucan could be extracted from brewers yeast with 60% purity- 60% purity for beta glucan is very practical. As of summer 2001 the oat products still haven't been able to match this price and strength of the yeast products.

You must remember the natural supplement industry can be as bad as any other since advertising and profits generally can be more important than helping people be healthier and living longer naturally. There are some wonderful, sincere and dedicated people in this industry, but they are definitely in the minority. You will see endless arguments that mushroom (the most expensive source of all) glucan is superior, or that yeast glucan is superior, or that oat glucan is superior. One company swears theirs is free of fat and protein which makes it superior! The consumer can get very confused as to which source is better and how much does one need to take and what price is fair.

Chemically we only need to be concerned that what we buy is a true 1,3-D-beta glucan. This means it is a basic "1,3" position on the glucose chain. Yeast and mushroom glucans are 1,3/1,6 positions while oat and barley glucans are 1,3/1,4 positions. It just doesn't make any difference folks- they are all true 1,3 glucans and basically they all have the same biological benefits. This was proven quite conclusively in 1997 at the University of Hamburg in Germany (Carbohydrate Research volume 297, pages 135-43). Dr. Kulicke and his cohorts concluded, "All glucans investigated regardless of molar mass and solution structure stimulate the investigated immunological measures more than a commercially available biomedical drug used for comparison." They discovered this after studying human blood monocytes for, "tumor necrosis factor alpha release activity". This basically means they measured real human blood to see how the glucans would help strengthen immune qualities and resist infection.

What are the major benefits of taking beta glucan? This nutrient benefits anyone who wants to be healthier, live longer, deal with the stress of modern society, be less allergenic, speed up healing and resist the dangerous microbes, bacteria and viruses that seem to be everywhere. As you saw in the contents, the major reason to take beta glucan is to enhance your immune system. If you have benign or malignant tumors it is a powerful adjuvant (which means to aid or help) to whatever else you are doing, whether it is taking chemotherapy or eating a macrobiotic diet. It is an effective way to lower cholesterol and triglycerides especially when used with other natural supplements. The effects on your skin- especially on your face- are dramatic and it should be a daily part of your skin care routine. It has been found to help regulate blood sugar levels especially in cases of diabetes. There are various other benefits such as protection from ionizing radiation that are discussed in chapter 6. Now that beta glucan is inexpensive and has come out of the scientific closet after all these years we will certainly see many more studies especially with real people to find new uses for this wondrous food extract.

How much should you take? Some studies used ridiculous amounts in test animals like 100 mg per kilogram. This equates to about 7,000 mg (7 grams!) in a human male. Interestingly enough they found no negative side effects even at such extreme doses. Generally people take 100 mg a day for immunity and cholesterol lowering. If you have a medical condition and want to add beta glucan to your repetoire you can take 200-500 mg a day. If I had, say, diabetes, cancer or another serious condition I would take up to 300 to 500 mg a day for at least a year and then drop down to a maintenance dose of the usual 100 mg.

Can you take this with prescription drugs and medication? Certainly! Of course you want to tell your doctor what you are doing. Beta glucan is merely a food extract we find abundantly in such foods as oatmeal and yeasted bread and has no known side effects at all even in very extreme doses. It has a Generally Recognized as Safe (GRAS) classification from the FDA. Actually it has been shown repeatedly to enhance the actions of many such drugs. For example, if you are taking an antibiotic it may well help the potency of it. If you are taking a cholesterol lowering drug it will probably help lower your cholesterol even further. If you are on diabetes medication it should potentiate that.

You may be wondering how beta glucan works so powerfully. It would be very presumptuous to think we understand that very well, but certain things are known. We have large white blood cells "macrophages" (i.e. great eaters) such as phagocytes, neutrophils and other such cells found in all the tissues of our bodies that literally devour bacteria, foreign cells, dead and dying cells, mutated cells and other negative invaders in our bloodstreams. They are the most important cells in our immune system. For example, natural killer (NK) cells eat the cancer and infected cells along with these. These important cells in our immune systems are activated and strengthened by beta

11

glucan, by means we don't yet truly understand. When you take a beta glucan supplement these immune cells are more active, more powerful and effective in attacking and consuming what doesn't belong in our systems.

What is the best kind to take? Barley derived beta glucan has never been offered because oats are a more economical source. Oat beta glucan is less popular than yeast because yeast derived is more concentrated and less expensive. Mushroom beta glucan is the most expensive of all and the worst choice for your money. Some manufacturers claim they use bakers yeast, but this seems rather unbelievable since brewers yeast is a much less expensive source. Millions of pounds of brewers yeast are discarded by the beer breweries every year and this is why brewers yeast beta glucan is the most economical choice as of the year 2001. What about allergies to yeast? Yeast, whether bakers of brewers, is one of the top ten allergenic foods known. Beta glucan, however, is so well extracted and only from the cell walls of the yeast that even at only 60% purity any allergenic proteins are probably completely removed or present in such small doses as to not affect you physically.

Chapter 2: Nature's Strongest Immunity Enhancer

You have heard about exotic, bioengineered supposed wonders of medical science like "interferon" for enhancing immunity that are priced out of the reach of any but the rich. The truth is that interferon has been an overtouted failure from the beginning, and that the strongest immunity enhancer on earth has been known about for over twenty years now. Nothing rivals beta glucan for immune enhancement. No substance on earth manmade or natural has the published studies to back it up like beta glucan does. In the following pages you will see the last fifteen years of published research to prove this to you. The many patents will not be included since so many studies are available.

At Tulane University in New Orleans in 1987 (International Journal of Immunopharmacology volume 9, pages 261-7), researchers showed that beta glucan enhanced the production of both interleukin-1 (IL-1) and interleukin-2 (IL-2) in rats. Their plasma levels of IL-1 and IL-2 were measured after this was given. They concluded, "Thus beta 1,3 glucan will enhance IL-1 and IL-2 production and elevations in lymphokine production can be maintained up to 12 days."

At the INRA research center in Touloose, France in 1989 (Annals of Veterinary Research volume 20, pages 165-73) fungal glucans were studied for their immunopotentiating activity in mice and the researchers said they, "favorably affect the non-specific host defense and cellular immune response in mice."

At Tokyo College Pharmacy in Japan much work was done over the years on glucans. In 1989 (International Journal of Immunopharmacology volume 11, pages 761-9) they gave oral glucan from mushrooms (Sclerotinia) to mice and found this, "enhanced the activities of both natural killer (NK) cells in the spleen and the lysosomal enzyme of peritoneal macrophages."

A very impressive study using malaria was done at Rangaraya Medical College in India in 1990 (Indian Journal of

Experimental Biology volume 28, pages 901-5). Malaria (Plasmodium berghi) was injected into mice and death was prevented in most of the ones receiving the glucan while the untreated ones died. They said, "The results suggest that glucan potentiated both limbs of immunity and both were involved in the host defense against malaria."

At the MacArthur Center for Tropical Diseases in Israel in 1991 (Parasite Immunology volume 13, pages 137-45) deadly Leishmania major germs were injected into mice. Some mice were given yeast beta glucan, which mitigated most of the effects of this devastating bacteria. They concluded, "The anti-Leishmania antibody titer of glucan treated mice was lower and their sera recognized fewer antigens than that of control Leishmania bearing mice."

At the famous Karolinska Institute in Stockholm a very good study was done in 1991 on real human natural killer (NK) cells (European Journal of Immunology volume 21, pages 1755-8). They used human NK cells which actually bind to the beta glucan and they concluded, "The function of NK cells was also potentiated by preincubation with beta glucan. The treatment increased the proportion of target-binding lymphocytes and of the damaged target cells in the conjugates." In plain English it made the NK cells more powerful and effective.

At the university of Californa at Davis in 1992 (International Journal of Immunopharmacology volume 14, pages 767-72) mice were studied for their immune responses. It was found that beta glucan was an excellent "adjuvant" which is an immune enhancer that augments immune response. The found, "glucan and lipovant present effective adjuvant alternative, to Freund's complete adjuvant and may be of value in immunization against visceral leishmaniasis" (Leishmania infantum was the bacteria they used in this experiment).

At the Tokyo College of Pharmacy in Hachioji in 1993 (Biology Pharmacy Bulletin volume 16, pages 414-9) mushroom beta glucan called OL-2 was studied on mice for their specific immune responses including white blood cells, tumor necrosis factor, bone marrow cells, colony stimulating factors and other parameters. They said, "These facts suggested that OL-2 could

14

enhance nonspecific host defense mechanisms by enhancing hematopoietic responses..." In other words in beta glucan gives nonspecific immune enhancement by various means.

At the Ustav Biofaktory in the Czech Republic in 1993 (Biopharm volume 3, pages 71-82) dairy cows were given yeast beta glucan in a double blind experiment. Various biological responses were measured and they found optimal doses to be given the cows to strengthen their immunity. In raising farm animals like cows, pigs, and sheep it is important to keep their immunity high so they will be resistant to disease. Beta glucan is an inexpensive way to insure the health of such animals.

At the Nippon Roche Research Center in Japan in 1994 (FEBS Letters volume 348, pages 27-32) researchers used a killer toxin called HM-1 for this experiment. They found that beta glucan interfered with the toxin action of HM-1. They reported, "Addition of HM-1 killer toxin with several kinds of oligosaccharides revealed that either beta 1,3 or beta 1,6 glucan block the cytocidal (toxic) action of HM-1 killer toxin..." Again, this shows that it does not matter whether the beta glucan is 1,3 which we are concerned with, or even the 1,6 configuration (which is also found in common foods) to be effective.

At Purdue University in Indiana in 1995 (Carbohydrate Polymers volume 28, pages 3-14) 1,3 beta glucan was studied for configuration and structure in relation to immunostimulant activity. They reported their findings that, "Immunopotentiation effected by binding of 1,3 beta glucan molecules or particles probably includes activation of cytotoxic macrophages, helper T cells, and NK cell, promotion of T Cell differentiation and activation of the alternative complement pathway." In simpler terms they feel that beta glucan works by assisting macrophages, T cells and NK cells basically.

At SRI International in California in 1995 (Advances in Experimental and Medical Biology volume 383, pages 13-22) scientists used beta glucan to enhance humoral (fluids like blood and lymph) and cell-mediated immune responses to viral proteins. They said, "Our studies in mice and rabbits demonstrated that co-administering viral protein with beta glucan produces immune responses of a higher magnitude than those elicited by the immunogens alone."

At the State Univeristy of Tennessee in 1996 (Proceedings-Beltwide Cotton Conference volume 1, pages 285-8) researchers were aware that "Glucans, isolated from natural sources, are known to stimulate humoral and cell-mediated immunity in humans and animals. It is now established that 1,3 beta glucans are recognized by macrophages and perhaps, neutrophils and NK cells via a 1,3 beta glucan specific receptor. Following receptor binding, glucan modulates macrophage cytokine expression." This simply means they understand the way glucans work is by binding to macophages, neutrophils and NK cells and making them more potent in their defense of the body.

At the James Quillen College of Medicine in Tennessee doctors published an overview of the immunology of beta glucan in 1997 (Mediators Inflammation volume 6, pages 247-50). "It is now established that 1,3 beta glucans area recognized by macrophages and perhaps neutrophils and natural killer cells via a 1,3 beta glucan specific receptor." Yes, these are some of the same doctors that attended the Beltwide Cotton Conference a year earlier; they now published a review in another journal.

A study from the University of Saskatchewan took place in 1997 (Microbiological Immunology volume 41, pages 991-8) with oat glucans they called OBG. OBG was tested for its ability to enhance non-specific resistance to a bacterial challenge in mice. Survival in mice challenged with deadly Staphylococcus aureus was enhanced by a single dose of OBG three days prior to the bacteria being administered. "These studies demonstated that OBG possesses immunomodulatory activities capable of stimulating immune functions both in vitro and in vivo." Staphylococcus is one of the most deadly of bacteria to mammals and for beta glucan to resist this is rather impressive medically.

Another study at the University of Saskatchewan in Canada in 1997 (International Journal of Parasitology volume 27, pages 329-37) oat beta glucan was studied in mice. The deadly Eimeria vermiformis bacteria was given to mice and their immune systems were suppressed with the toxic drug dexamethasone. The immuosuppressed mice who received no beta glucan showed severe symptoms of disease and a 50% mortality, while minimal symptoms and no mortality occurred in the beta glucan treated groups. There was no mortality when simply given beta glucan! They summarized the results that beta glucan treatment strongly increased the resistance to Eimeria infection even when the immune system was chemically suppressed.

In 1998 the people at the University of Saskatchewan again studied OBG and this time on the deadly Eimeria vermiformis bacteria. Oat beta glucan given to mice raised their levels of serum Igs (immunoglobulins) and antigen-specific Igs (specialized immunoglobulins). One group was not given any glucan and the other group was before both groups were infected with the Eimeria. They said, "OBG appeared to up-regulate immune mechanisms and provide enhanced resistance against Eimerian coccidiosis in mice." Again glucans saved mammals from death by a most deadly bacteria.

At the National Hospital in Oslo in 1998 (Scandinavian Journal of Immunology volume 47, pages 548-53) more scientists studied mice. This time they were given beta glucan before being infected with the deadly Mycobacterium bovis bacteria. Mice treated with the beta glucan showed significantly lower numbers of bacteria in their bodies and especially in their spleens and livers. They said, "The results suggest that beta glucan has a protective effect against Mycobacterium bovis infection in susceptible mice."

At the Slovak Academy of Sciences in Bratislava in 1999 (Carbohydrate Polymers, vol. 38, p.247-53) doctors studied beta glucans from both yeast and fungus (Aspergillus) to see if they would stimulate immunity using live cells and sophisticated FTIR spectroscopy. They concluded that, "It has been found that the derivatives prepared reveal high mitogenic and comitogenic activities, as well as radioprotective and antimutagenic effects. "In other words it stimulates immunity in four basic different ways."

Yet again at the University of Saskatchewan in 1999 (Canadian Journal of Veterinary Research vol. 63, pages 262-8) scientists studied beta glucan but this time on beef steers. They used the stand "OBG" extract from oats. They got varied results with different groups but the most interesting result was when the steers had they immune systems suppressed with dexamethasone the glucan overcame this very effectively. Very sophisticated parameters were measured including serum antibody responses, serum IgG (immunoglobin G) levels, blastogenic responses of blood lymphocytes, differential blood leukocytes as well as iron and zinc levels in the blood. They said, "When cells or animals were treated with dexamethasone, OBG significantly restored some of the specific and non-specific immune parameters studied."

At the National Institute of Public Health in Oslo in 2000 (FEMS Immunology Medical Microbiology volume 27, pages 111-6) doctors studied fungal beta glucan against deadly Strepococcus pneumoniae, a potent pneumonia strain. They called their beta glucan extract "SSG". They said, "The data demonstrate that SSG administered systemically protects against pneumococcal infection in mice." Of course you can't ethically give one group of humans beta glucan and not to another group and then infect them both with deadly pneumonia, but there is no reason to doubt that this would also protect humans just as well.

Over twenty clinical studies done at well known research facilities over the world and published in various scientific journals should convince you this is the most potent immune potentiating substance known to science. It is safe, natural, effective and inexpensive with no know side effects.

Chapter 3: Tumors – Benign and Malignant

Of all the many studies on the various powers of beta glucan it was surprising how many concerned tumors and cancer. It is not just macrophages here that attack tumors but also natural killer cells (NK), killer T cells, lymphokines and interleukin-1 and – 2. All these scientific terms just refer to the various processes we have to attack tumor cells and remove them from our bodies. There are literally dozens of studies on the anti-tumor properties of beta glucan just in the last fifteen years, and we'll try to mention as many as possible. Journal references will not be given for simplicity and brevity here. Is what stood out especially in all these is that the beta glucan came from a great variety of sources, but they were all true 1,3 beta glucans whether from oats, barley, yeast, mushrooms or a great variety of various fungi. Again, this shows all basic true 1,3 beta glucans have the same general power to fight and destroy tumors in our bodies.

At Kobe Women's College in Japan maitake mushroom (Grifola frondosa) beta glucan showed clear anti-tumor effect against both MM-46 and IMC carcinomas (these simply refer to the type of cancer strains) in mice. Again at the Kobe Women's College beta glucan from Cochliobolus mushroom inhibited the growth of Sarcoma 180 (the most popular strain) solid tumors in mice. At the Study Center for Nuclear Energy in Belgium Lentinus mushroom (Lentinus edodes) beta glucan arrested lymphoma cells in the blood of mice.

At the Tokyo College of Pharmacy in Japan maitake beta glucan had anti-tumor activity against MM-46 and "syngenic" tumors in general. Again, at the Tokyo College of Pharmacy beta glucan from Sclerotinia mushroom was shown to be effective against Sarcoma 180 solid tumors in mice. They called this extract "SSG" and said, "SSG is a useful antitumor glucan which modifies biological responses." A third study at this college with SSG extract found more proof of antitumor activity. A fourth study at this college used the same SSG extract but this time against pulmonary metastasis or lung cancer using Lewis lung carcinoma implanted cells in mice. In just 10 days the lung cancer cells were inhibited even when the SSG was simply placed in their daily feed. A fifth study used the same "OL" extract from Omphalia or "leiwan" mushroom and said, "OL-2 showed characteristic features regarding its physiochemical properties and antitumor activity."

At the University of Regensburg in Germany beta glucan extracted from Phytophthora mushrooms was effective against Sarcoma 180 solid tumors in mice. Again, at the University of Regensburg beta glucans were taken from various fungi and used successfully again Sarcoma 180 solid tumors in mice. They found that all were very potent in this regardless of the source. Tumor weights were reduced 72 to 99% in only 30 days with no other treatments! A third study was done here using an extract of the Glomerella mushroom with the impressive result that 100% of both Sarcoma I80 and MC.SC-1 (another basic cancer strain) fibrosarcoma tumors were inhibited. They stressed, "that a highly ordered structure of the glucan is not essential for the antitumor activity." A review of beta glucans in general was done in Germany at Georg-August University. This review studied the various sources, structures, effects on the immune system and clinical application for their extensive antitumor properties.

At the Research Institute for Life Sciences in Japan Cordyceps mushroom beta glucan was studied for antitumor activity and the structure compared for biological response. As usual the 1,3 configuration was the basic consideration making it a true beta glucan. Another study with lung cancer cells was done at the world famous Mayo Clinic in Minnesota. In only I4 days the lung cancer growth was measurably inhibited and the mice given the beta glucan were alive while the untreated mice were dying.

At Osaka City University in Japan the well known reishi mushroom (Ganoderma lucidum) was used as a source for beta glucan and tested for antitumor activity. As usual, the researchers stressed the basic true 1,3 backbone structure and not the 1,4 or 1,6 branching. They found this to be very powerful against Sarcoma 180 solid tumors in mice. Nearby at the University of Osaka a review was done complete with 54 different references on the many studies done on antitumor activity, the structures, mechanisms of action and clinical applications.

Poria cocos is a classic Chinese mushroom that has been used in their herbal tradition for many centuries. It is also known as hoelen or fu ling. At the University of Wuhan in China beta glucan was extracted from Poria and studied to see how it inhibited both Sarcoma 180 and Ehrlich (another strain) carcinoma. They were very successful in treating both of these in mice.

At the University of Shizuoka in Japan beta glucan from reishi, maitake and plain agaricus (common edible) mushrooms were all compared for antitumor activity. The standard procedure of using mice with implanted Sarcoma 180 solid tumors was used for consistency and the usual success was found. A second study at this university this time used an extract from Polyporus mushrooms for their source of beta glucan. They found the same basic antitumor power in this mushroom as well.

At the Tokyo Metropolitan Research Lab in Japan beta glucan was extracted from Omphalia lapidescens fungi, which they called "OL" extracts. They compared the various structures of the extracts and used them in Sarcoma 180 solid tumors in mice and found strong antitumor activity regardless of the branching as long at the basic structure was 1,3 configuration. A second study at this laboratory used the same OL extracts and found more proof of antitumor activity using the same mice and same cancer strain.

The Japanese government granted patent #JP 03,133,934 in 1991 for using Polyphorus confluens mushroom beta glucan for antitumor activity in general due to the studies that were done on animals proving its value repeatedly. The international patent authority approved WO 98 27,992 in 1998 for Agaricus blazei (common edible) mushroom beta glucan for it's general antitumor effects especially against solid cancers. The Japanese government later granted patent #JP10 287,284 in 1998 for using beta glucan generally which inhibits tumor growth by activating natural killer cells.

At Joseph Fourier University in France beta glucan from Laetisaria (a Basidiomycete mushroom) was studied in the usual Sarcoma 180 solid tumors in mice. "The polysaccharide strongly inhibited tumor growth with an inhibition ratio of almost 100%." To have this kind of success is incredible.

At the National Cancer Institute Research Center in Japan researchers used an extract of the fungus Hypsizigus marmoreus for their beta glucan against both Sarcoma 180 and the syngenic Meth A fibrosarcoma (another strain). They found this to be effective for both but especially for the Sarcoma 180 malignancy. At Christian-Albrechts University in Germany an extract of the Pythium mushroom was used as the source of beta glucan. They said that a mere hot water extract, "exhibited strong activity against Sarcoma 180 in CD-1 (a specific type of) mice."

At the Tokyo University Pharmacy three different kinds of fungal glucans were used for a total of ten weeks (five weeks before implanting tumors and five weeks after) in mice to effectively inhibit Sarcoma 180 solid tumors. At the University of Louisville in Kentucky a review with multiple references was done on the studies of beta glucan on tumors and cancer. This is written in very sophisticated and scientific terms but in plain English they suggest using beta glucan as cancer therapy in humans in 1999 due to the many years of animal studies. Doctors like this deserve a lot of credit, but the vast majority of physicians are not going to use inexpensive, natural remedies no matter how well they work for cancer or any other disease.

At the Eishogen Research Center in Japan mushroom glucan "showed marked antitumor activities against Sarcoma 180" in mice. Peritoneal macrophages multiplied strongly. There is no reason this won't show the same results in humans when such studies are finally done and published.

In these many studies you can see that beta glucan works regardless of where it is found and what source is used. After almost two decades overwhelming proof with animal studies it is time to use beta glucan on real people in clinical studies. Any individual can choose to use beta glucan with traditional medical treatments or with other natural healing methods as diet, supplements, hormone balancing, exercise and fasting. We still need human studies published in the medical journals to prove objectively that this is something that should be considered by anyone with benign or malignant tumors and cancerous growths.

Chapter 4: Lower Your Cholesterol

It has been well known to scientists for over two decades now that beta glucan has very strong cholesterol and triglyceride lowering properties. Many of these studies were done on test animals for a long time before humans were used. This is the usual progression of events in clinical studies to make sure a supplement actually works and is safe. Additionally animal studies are much less expensive to perform.

At the Technical Research Institute in Kawagoe, Japan (Nippon Eiyo Shokuryo 44 (1991) p. 455-60) obese rats with high cholesterol were given both oat and barley beta glucan to effectively lower their cholesterol levels. Another study done there (Journal of Nutritional Science and Vitaminology 40 (1994) p. 213-17) more rats were given oat and barley beta glucan and some were given guar gum. All were effective in improving blood lipid profiles. At the University of California in Davis (Journal of Food Science 60 (1995) p. 558-60) oat beta glucan was given to hypercholesteremic rats and lowered their levels in only four weeks by adding it to their feed. At the Montana Agricultural Station in Bozeman (Nutrition Research 17 (1997) p. 77-88) hamsters were fed barley beta glucan in a double blind study and their cholesterol was lowered within 30 days. At the Technical Research Center in Espoo, Finland (Cereal Chemistry 69 (1992) p. 647-53) more rats with high cholesterol were given oat beta glucan to successfully lower their cholesterol. Another study there (British Journal of Nutrition 70 (1993) p. 767-76) more rats with high cholesterol were given oat beta glucan in a classic double blind study where not even the scientists knew which rats were getting the supplement. Not only did the oat supplement lower their cholesterol but raised their desirable high density cholesterol levels as well. At the West Research Center in Albany, California (Cereral Chemistry 70 (1993) p. 435-40) hamsters with high cholesterol were given oat and barley beta glucan to lower their blood lipids in only 21 days.

The human studies leave no doubt that what was shown with animals is equally effective on real people. At Syracuse University in New York (Journal of the American Dietary Association 90 (1990) p. 223-9) 71 men and women with hypercholesteremia were given various combinations of low fat diets with and without oat beta glucan supplements. The people not only lowered their cholesterol up to 17% but most all of them raised their levels of beneficial high density cholesterol. This shows the power of using better food choices along with your supplements.

At Harvard Medical School in Massachusetts (Critical Reviews in Food Science and Nutrition 39 (1999), p. 189-202) doctors found that both oat and yeast derived beta glucans lowered serum cholesterol levels without any change in diet or exercise. There was no use of drugs, which you would expect at a school of medicine. In their words, "In addition to decreasing the intake of total fat, saturated fat and dietary cholesterol, blood serum cholesterol can be further decreased by dietary fiber, especially from sources rich in beta glucan such as oats and yeast." They do very much suggest low fat diets with little animal fat or cholesterol to their credit. Doctors like this deserve a lot of praise for studying natural ways and natural supplements to cure disease.

At the University of Massachusetts (American Journal of Clinical Nutrition 70, 1999, p. 208-12) researchers studied obese men with high cholesterol levels. They gave them yeast based beta glucan but made no changes in their diet or exercise. In only eight weeks cholesterol had fallen 8% and their harmful low density cholesterol levels had also fallen 8%. They summarized their findings, "Thus, the yeast derived beta glucan fiber lowered the total cholesterol concentrations and was well tolerated".

At the United States Human Nutrition Research Center in Maryland (Journal of Nutrition and Biochemistry 8, (1997) p. 497-501) people were given oat extracts high in beta glucan content and lowered their blood fats with no change in diet or exercise. They studied these people further and found some rather remarkable beneficial changes in their metabolism after just a few weeks on beta glucan supplements. For one thing they found their dietary fat was not oxidized as much as usual which is desirable. New benefits of this are constantly being discovered.

Again at the Human Nutrition Center (Journal of the American College of Nutrition 16 (1997) p. 46-51) men and women with high blood lipid levels were given oat extracts high in beta glucan. After only five weeks the groups were switched and those previously getting the oat extract received only the typical American high fat diet everyone was maintained on. At the end of the study it was shown that when each group got the beta glucan both their total cholesterol levels and low density cholesterol levels decreased significantly. In their words, "A significant dose response due to beta glucan concentration in the oat extract was observed in the total cholesterol levels." When you have such thorough double blind studies at prestigious research centers where people are given a high fat diet with no exercise, there is no doubt about the powerful effects of beta glucan on real people with high blood fat levelson less than desirable diets.

At Industrial Research Limited in New Zealand (Carbohydrate Polymers 29 (1996) p. 7-10) researchers used barley derived glucan to try and discover the actual metabolic mechanisms by which it lowered blood fats. They wanted to understand just beta glucan affects the various organs of the body to eliminate blood fats rather than let them build up. They first discovered that it increased the secretion of bile acids from the gall bladder. These bile acids are important in keeping cholesterol and triglycerides at healthy levels. They used high sophisticated NMR (nuclear magnetic resonance) techniques and found the bile acid process was only part of the story and the mechanism is much more complicated than mere enhanced gall bladder activity. This shows the more we learn the less we know and the important thing is that beta glucan is a powerful normalizer of blood fats and we may never clearly understand the mechanisms by which it works.

At the University of Lund in Sweden (Annals of Nutrition and Metabolism 43 (1999) p. 301-9) mildly hypercholesteremic men and women were given oat milk, which was high in beta glucan content in their diets for five weeks. This was a classic double blind study and half of the men got rice milk, which contains no beta glucan. The men drinking the oat milk lowered

25

their total cholesterol as well as their low density cholesterol levels while the men drinking the rice milk did not. They said, "It is concluded that oat milk has cholesterol reducing properties."

Worldwide studies like this on real people in research clinics and hospitals leave no doubt that beta glucan is a safe, effective, proven, powerful and inexpensive way to lower cholesterol and improve blood lipid profiles. There is every reason to use natural methods like this rather than dangerous, expensive drugs with serious side effects. One of these statin drugs was just removed from the market after too many people died after taking it. Is there any reason to believe the others are any safer? Yet most people have never even heard of beta glucan much less take it every day. Most drug stores, health food stores and vitamin companies don't even sell it and most of the brands offered are either weak and/or overpriced.

You can read my book "Lower Your Cholesterol without Drugs". In it the "cornerstone" program for reducing cholesterol includes five different natural supplements. In addition to 100 mg of beta glucan you can take flax oil, beta sitosterol, soy isoflavones and guggul gum. Take one or two one gram capsules of flax oil instead of fish oil supplements. Keep these in your refrigerator. Beta-sitosterol is an extract of sugar cane pulp or soybeans and can be found in some vitamin catalogs or on a search of the Internet. Take 300 mg of mixed sterols a day and do not use the margarines or salad dressings with soy sterols since they are expensive and full of fat. Soy isoflavones are a very important part of this program and you only need 40 mg a day of genestein and daidzein. You realistically cannot get enough isoflavones from eating soy foods, so taking a good supplement is the most practical way to do this. The last supplement is guggul gum, which is an Ayurvedic herb extracted from the Commiphora tree. Take 250 mg of a reliable supplement with 10% sterones to give you 25 mg of actual sterones per day. If you take these five "cornerstone" supplements you can even lower genetically high cholesterol levels without diet or exercise. With better food choices and simply walking every day your improvements can be really dramatic. Remember that natural health means a natural lifestyle and especially a natural diet.

Chapter 5: Rejuvenate Your Skin

Beta glucan has very powerful topical effects on your skin especially on your face. This has been known about for over fifteen years now, but no one has put out a cream with realistic amounts of beta glucan until very recently. This author put out a fine cream with one quarter of 1% oat derived beta glucan back in 1994. This was taken to the largest U.S. natural food and drug trade shows but was never commercially successful. The reason it wasn't a full one per cent cream was due to the gumminess of the oat beta glucan. This was due to the high cost and low percent of the raw beta glucan until about 1999. It is still very difficult to find a REAL beta glucan cream with one percent oat or yeast glucans. If you will search the Internet you will find one or two. Make sure they clearly state their creams contain at least one per cent (600 mg per 2 ounce jar). If they refuse to state how much or contain less than that, don't buy it. Back in 1987 a beta glucan cream was put out from yeast and heavily promoted with magazine ads but it contained a useless 10 mg (one thirtieth on one percent!) of yeast glucans per ounce. This was chemically and biologically useless and, of course, people got no benefits from it. Finally in 2001 for the first time you can find this due to the wonders of the Internet and the advancement in extraction technology.

We have already spoken of macrophages. Macrophages are in your skin and are activated by topical beta glucan just as the internal macrophages are. Our skin is not just a covering for our body- it is the largest organ of the body and the most important organ for our immune systems. The outer layer or epidermis contains about five per cent macrophages. These cells stop the growth of dangerous microbes and produce something called "epidermal growth factor" which stimulates renewal of skin cells.

Most of the studies done on topical uses have been done by private cosmetic and pharmaceutical companies and not published. They realize the profit potential here and want to patent and protect any discoveries they make. Therefore most of this chapter depends on patents they have registered. You'll see in the following studies that some of the largest cosmetic companies in the world are involved in this. We need more human studies on topical uses especially for wound healing and reducing aging and wrinkles in the skin. Until we get those studies just use a good beta glucan cream on your face for a year and see if you get the results you want.

In 1987 Bio Bi Daimaru Company in Japan was given patent #JP62,205,008 for a beta glucan cream from Aureobacidium. In 1991 Kanebo Limited in Japan was granted patent #JP 03,167,109 for their beta glucan cream from Macrophomopsis species. In 1992 Ichimaru Pharcos K.K. Company in Japan was granted patent #JP 04 59,715 for their beta glucan cream extracted from Euglena. In 1996 Noevir K.K. Company in Japan was granted patent #JP 08,291,01 for their beta glucan from any source.

There is a class of patents granted in the European Union called PCT International patents. The famous and huge conglomerate Ciba-Geigy A.G. Corporation was granted WO 95 22,310 patent in 1994 for a beta glucan cream containing "0.05% to 3.0%" glucans from Schizophylllium species. 0.05% is a mere one twentieth of one per cent so let's hope Ciba-Geigy uses at least I% in whatever cream they eventually put out as it is not on the market as of 2001. That such a large corporation has researched and patented a beta glucan is prima facie proof of its value. Another PCT patent was granted in France in 1996 #WO 96 28,008 for "controlling skin ageing and/or increasing skin elasticity". At the famous ROC Corporation who has been promoting retinol creams worldwide they were granted WO 98 17,246 in 1996 for a beta glucan cream. They only call for a 0.5% (half of one percent) beta glucan from unspecified sources but at least this is reasonable. The very successful Shaklee international multilevel marketing corporation was granted WO 99 33,439 in 1999 and then granted a United States patent as well for their beta glucan cream. They claim that their cream "increases the cellular viability of epidermal cells", and that it "decreases the production of inflammatory mediators" as well as "protecting the skin from the adverse effects of UV radiation". This is a successful company that knows what it is doing and would not spend the time and money on beta glucan cream if they didn't have good reason to see it as a major success. The even larger

28

firm of S.C. Johnson and Company was granted WO99 27,904 in 1999. An international corporation this large would not invest their time and money into patenting something unless they had very good research to show its value. Another very big international player is the Novogen Research Limited in Australia. They were granted WO99 36,050 in 1999 for their glucan cream. They claim their product "protects the skin from UV induced erythema, photoaging, and premalignant and malignant skin cancers." These are obviously strong claims to be granted in a PCT patent. The very successful Henkel Kommanditgesellschaft Corporation in Germany was granted WO98 40,082 in 1998 for their therapeutic glucan cream. They claimed, "These substances strengthen the immune system of the skin, counteract wrinkling and can be used to prevent scaling and psoriasis." Rather impressive claims obviously. Brennen Medical Incorporated was granted WO99 21,531 in 1999 for "healing treatment of burns and wounds and scarring therefrom". This shows the healing power for people who have been seriously hurt and want to heal faster and avoid scars.

At Alpha-Beta Technology, Incorporated in the U.S. a patent was granted in 1996 #5,488,040 for a beta glucan cream. This was a very sophisticated and complete patent. They claimed "Topical application of a solution of this glucan promoted wound healing in mice and eliminated experimental wound infection with Stapholococcus aureus." Staph infections are notorious for their hard to treat and deadly nature. This patent continued in great deal and medical language to explain the mechanisms of healing.

The German government granted patent DE 19,901,270 in 1999 to the Pacific Group of South Korea for their therapeutic glucan cream, which they said is used, "as an active component in a compound for external application that can delay skin changes and can heal and brighten skin." The famous Swiss Ciba Specialty Chemicals division of Ciba-Geigy Corporation was granted European patent EP 875,244 in 1997 for their glucan cream but did not make specific claims for its use surprisingly.

In 1995 a study was published in the trade journal Cosmetics and Toiletries (Italy) volume 16, pages 54-6. They actually used human subjects to apply their beta glucan cream to from yeast. They found clear antiaging properties, maintenance of cell integrity, improved skin metabolic function and protection

29

against photoaging (sun damage). We need more studies like this on real human subjects. In 1998 a second study was published from the Canadian company Canamino who was leading the world in beta glucan technology and application at the time (Cosmetics and Toiletries volume 113, pages 45-50). They use oat derived glucans to repair of skin from environmental damage from UV radiation, pollution, smoke, bacteria and free radicals.

In the Slovakian journal Farmacie Obzor in 1997 volume 66, pages 119-23 researchers used beta glucan from Pleurotus mushrooms. They applied a solution of this topically to mice and found "significant stimulation of defense mechanisms....increased phagocyte activity....higher microbiological activity of peritoneal macrophages and other very powerful effects. This was a very well done and very impressive study proving the specific mechanisms on the skin of live mice.

In 1997 the trade digest SOFW Journal in Germany two articles were published in the 123rd volume (pages 535-8 and 542-6). The first one was from Mibelle A.B. Biochemistry in Switzerland who used topical glucan to protect skin from UV radiation and to promote the growth of keratinocytes (growth cells) in humans and enhanced the immune system of the skin generally. The second one was from Verlag fur Chemische Industrie in Germany. They extracted 1,3 beta glucans from a variety of sources including yeast and various mushroom and fungi. They found these to be effective regardless of the source in topical preparations for human skin to protect and regenerate the cells.

In the trade publication International Journal of Cosmetic Science in 1998 (volume 20, page 79-86) Mibelle AG Cosmetics in Switzerland studied glucan creams on people to report the effects. They said these "are involved in the activation of the body's natural defense systems and in the acceleration of the skin's wound healing processes. In placebo controlled studies on real people they proved various benefits including protecting the skin from UV sun damage.

You'll see many more of these types of studies in the future.

Chapter 6: Other Benefits of Beta Glucan

There are many other health benefits from taking beta glucan daily as a supplement in addition to what we have already covered. There will be many more discovered as time goes on. Right now we have studies on such areas as diabetes and blood sugar, ulcers, the qualities of our blood, digestion of our food, protection from radiation and other positive effects on our bodies.

The most impressive of these is the effect on our blood sugar levels and diabetes. If you have diabetes you should consider taking a strong dose of at least 200 mg a day of beta glucan for a year and see if there is any improvement. You can also take all fruit, fruit juice, dried fruit and any sweetener out of your diet including honey, molasses and maple syrup. Sugar is sugar.

In 1989 at the University of Matsuyama in Japan (Horumon to Rinsho volume 37, pages 533-6) doctors studied the effect on giving beta glucan to insulin dependent (IDDM) Brattleboro rats. They found that this inhibited diabetes mellitus and insulinitis. This also increased the leucocyte count in their blood.

At the University of Laval in Quebec doctors studied oat glucan on the effects on insulinemia and glycemia in Sprague-Dawley rats. First of all they found that giving them the beta glucan reduced their food intake. Then they verified that glucose metabolism was improved generally which they called a "hypoinsulinic action" which means their insulin was more effective in controlling the blood levels of glucose (blood sugar). Further it was discovered that digestive tract function was improved and this was clearly connected to the improvement in glucose metabolism.

At Ehime University in Japan in 1992 (Diabetes Research and Clinical Practice, volume 17, pages 75-9) doctors again studied rats with diabetes and insulinitis. The diabetes rate was lowered from 43.3% to only 6.7% simply by giving them mushroom beta glucan (Lentinus edodes). The insulinitis rate was lowered from 82.4% to only 26.3% the same way. Most all of the rats stayed free from diabetes even when the supplement was discontinued which shows this was not merely a palliative but had healed them. Again their blood leucocytes were increased making their blood healthier. They concluded, "These data indicate that immunopotentiators could modulate the autoimmune mechanisms directed to pancreatic islets and inhibit the development of diabetes in Brattleboro rats."

At the University of Mitahora-Higashi in Japan in 1994 (Carbohydrate Research volume 251, pages 81-7) researchers studied diabetic mice by giving them mushroom (Agrocybe) beta glucan. This was simply extracted with hot water and called AG-HN1. They concluded, "AG-HN1 showed a remarkable hypoglycemic activity in both normal and streptozotocin-induced diabetic mice by i.p. administration (injection)." It is interesting that they lowered the plasma glucose levels of both diabetic AND normal mice. To lower the blood sugar of normal animals with a natural supplement is rather amazing to say the least. References were given as to other studies that showed hypoglycemic activity of beta glucan.

You might be asking yourself if anyone bothered to take such valuable research into human research? At the Centre for Food and Animal Research in Canada in 1994 (Carbohydrate Polymers volume 25, pages 331-6) this was finally done. A review was published with a full 39 references on the ability of oat glucan to moderate the postprandial (after meal) blood glucose and insulin response in humans. Since that time this author has been unable to find any other human studies on this. The animal research is clear and anyone with a blood sugar metabolism disorder should consider trying this. The effects on low blood sugar (hypoglycemia) have not been addressed unfortunately.

Gastric ulcers are rather much of an epidemic in Western society. Beta glucan has shown potential to heal these ulcers since it has such a strong effect on the digestive system in general. In 1993 at Koshien University in Japan (Koshien Daigaku Kiyo volume 19, pages 89-95) studies were done with barley beta glucan on rats. They induced ulcers by water immersion stress over time and found that by simply feeding them barley flour high in beta glucan they were very effectively protected from getting stress ulcers. Again, at Koshien University in the same journal later in 1996 (volume 23, pages 11-17) more rats were induced to get ulcers by water immersion and more barley derived glucan was given to them in their diets. Again, a strong protective effect was found. A third study at this university in the same journal (volume 26, pages 19-24) only this time with oat derived glucan with the same effects.

We have seen in some of the studies just mentioned that blood parameters were improved as a side effect of other benefits. The fact that beta glucan can improve the very quality of our blood is of great importance obviously.

At the Tokyo College of Pharmacy in 1990 (Pharmacobio-Dynamics volume 3, pages 525-32) researchers studied the effects of mushroom (Grifola) beta glucan on human plasma. Proper blood clotting is one of the basic qualities of our circulatory system. If blood clots too much you end up with clumping that causes strokes and other problems. If there is insufficient clotting you can't stop internal or external bleeding. It was found that beta glucan normalized clotting so this should not affect people on blood thinners like coumarin. The researchers found that beta glucan enhanced the ability of blood to clot normally, to bind with fibrinogen (which is a desirable trait) and to "increase the local concentration of the clotting system by steric exclusion." This was an excellent eight page study complete with twenty-six published references at one of Japan's top universities.

At Brigham Women's Hospital in Boston in 1994 (Immunology volume 81, pages 96-102) yeast glucans were again studied for their effect on human blood. The doctors said, "glucocorticoids enhance monocyte functions mediated by beta glucan receptors, and this stimulation is dependent on proteins that are newly synthesized during culture." This means that the glucan enhanced the functions of the monocytes and improved the blood metabolism in general.

United States patent 5,488,040 was granted in 1996 to Alpha-Beta Technology for the improvement of blood metabolism. They claimed that yeast beta glucan stimulates platelet production in human blood. They made other claims as to improving the metabolism of blood including tumor necrosis factor stimulation, phagocytes, stimulation of cytokines and general immunology. They also claimed that topical application "promoted wound healing" and "eliminated experimental wound infection with Staphalococcus aureus." Staph infection is known to be among the worst known bacteria and hardest to resist.

We saw in the discussion of diabetes that digestion is improved in test animals by giving them beta glucan. More specific studies were done to verify this. In 1995 in the Journal of Nutrition (volume 125, pages 947-55) barley glucan was given to chickens. Poultry farming is a very important industry in the United States and raising healthy chickens profitably is literally a multi billion dollar business. At the Department of Animal Nutrition in Spain it was found that feeding the chickens barley glucan improved their digestive enzymes and they ate less and gained less weight. Now this is not good news for the poultry industry and they want the broilers to gain as much weight as possible as quickly as possible for more profit. This is good news for both healthy chickens and humans in that you would eat less and gain less weight on less food.

PCT patent WO98 26,787 was granted in 1998 to the very large firm Gist-Brocades in Australia for the improvement of intestinal health with beta glucan. They discovered very strong improvement in digestion of test animals by adding this to their daily feed. These improvements included enhancing the amount of important Lactobacillus organisms especially. This is called a "probiotic effect" and means the healthy bacteria in our intestines, which are responsible for digesting our food, are increased. The Lactobacillus strain is the most important of these digestive bacteria, and are very deficient in most Western cultures because of our diets and lifestyles.

The Japanese government granted patent JP 08,157,377 in 1996 for using beta glucan to control diarrhea. They used mushroom (Aureobasidium) glucan to effectively control diarrhea especially for raising commercial animals like cows and pigs.

Another PCT patent was issued in 1992 WO94 04,136 for irritable bowel syndrome, including diarrhea and constipation in humans. This shows that many companies around the world realize the value of beta glucan in many health conditions and are busy trying to patent their particular product. Every year you will see more and more such patents.

It is almost impossible to protect people from the effects of radioactive contamination. When a nuclear reactor spews uranium or plutonium mist into the air, water and soil it contaminates people, animals and plants. Since there is no concentrated nuclear radiation in nature this is not a natural condition and the usual natural means of cure are rarely effective. Beta glucan has been shown to be effective in resisting the effects of such nuclear damage. In Belgium at the Center for Nuclear Energy in 1988 (Pharmacology Therapy volume 39, pages 255-9) researchers found that yeast beta glucan protected mice against the effects of x-radiation. When mice were irradiated and given beta glucan supplements their bone marrow stem cells resisted the effects and they had a much higher survival rate than the mice not given the supplements. At the same facility in Belgium in the same journal (pages 189-93) they also studied mice given whole body irradiation with and without beta glucan supplementation. They studied their general health including gastrointestinal function and blood parameters and found that the supplemented mice successfully resisted the radiation much more than the unsupplemented mice. At the Armed Forces Radiobiological Research Institute in Maryland in 1988 mice were irradiated and given a variety of supplements to see which protected them the most. The beta glucan supplements were most effective and the mice were analyzed for other metabolic functions. They concluded, "the results indicate the potential use of immunomodulators for protection against acute radiation injury..." At the Czech Academy of Science in 1991 radioprotective benefits of glucans were again studied on mice. They found increased recovery and increased survival in the mice given the supplements (Folia Biologica volume 37, pages 117-24).

At the University of Bratislava in Slovakia in 1986 (Methods and Findings of Experiemental and Clinical Pharmacology volume 8, pages 163-6) it was shown that yeast beta glucan increased the macrophage activity of guinea pigs. It was also shown that superoxide activity was increased. Superoxide dismutase (SOD) is one of the basic antioxidant enzymes we have that fight free radicals. SOD falls as we age and free radicals become much more effective and harmful. They said, "Macrophages from

35

guinea pigs treated with glucans exerted an increased ability to reduce INT and to produce superoxide."

At the Laboratory for Biological and Cellular Molecules in France in 1989 (Reproduction and Nutritional Development volume 29, pages 139-46) yeast beta glucan was given to sheep as well as barley beta glucan. They found that this stimulated hormone secretion especially valuable growth hormone. They found that this actually increased milk production in the ewes making them more valuable and healthier at the same time. It is very difficult to increase the production of growth hormone and this is basic to how long we live and how healthy we are.

At the famous Mayo Clinic in Minnesota in 1993 (Immunological Letters volume 37, pages 19-25) doctors found that tumor necrosis factor activity was enhanced in test animals by yeast beta glucan. Tumor necrosis factor is a potent cytokine or protein that is necessary to resist and kill and both benign and malignant tumor cells. This prevented the death of animals challenged with deadly bacteria. They said, "The authors therefore hypothesized that beta glucan might regulate TNF (tumor necrosis factor) secretion from macrophages in response to liposaccharide (LPS)." They went on to say that, "these data suggest an immunomodulatory role of beta glucan which may explain both the TNF stimulating and inhibited effects of fungal beta glucans during infection." At the Tokyo College Pharmacy that has been doing so much research on glucans they also studied TNF in 1995 (Biology and Pharmacy Bulletin volume 18, pages 126-33). Mushroom (Grifola) glucan was given to mice and elevated the LPS, which stimulated TNF production. This occurred within two hours and lasted a full three weeks. More verification of the means by which glucans fight tumors.

This short list of benefits is only the beginning. More and more we'll discover new benefits for taking this wondrous substance that is found in our everyday food. This should be one of the most important supplements you take for a long and healthy life.

OTHER BOOKS AVAILABLE FROM SAFE GOODS

The Natural Prostate Cure	$ 6.95 US $10.95 CAN
No More Horse Estrogen!	$ 7.95 US $11.95 CAN
Lower Cholesterol Without Drugs	$ 6.95 US $10.95 CAN
The Secrets of Staying Young	$ 9.95 US $14.95 CAN
Natural Anti-Aging Skin Care	$ 4.95 US $ 7.95 CAN
The High Performance Diet	$ 7.95 US $ 11.95 CAN
Curing Allergies with Visual Imagery	$ 14.95 US $ 22.95 CAN
Self-Care Anywhere	$19.95 US $29.95 CAN
Kid's – First: Health with No Interference	$12.95 US $19.95 CAN
Cell Towers: Wireless Convenience or Environmental Hazard?	$ 19.95 US $ 29.95 CAN

US (888) NATURE-1 (628-8731)   CAN (877) 742-7078
M/C VISA AMEX add $4.00 ea for shipping

Safe Goods/New Century Publishing 2000
US: PO Box 36, E. Canaan, CT 06024
CAN: 60 Bullock Dr., Unit 6, Markham, ON L3P 3P2